Cancer Has Nothing On Me

by Valorie R. Carney

Contents

Dedication

Chapter 1 – In The Beginning

Chapter 2 – When God Meets You

Chapter 3 – Why Again?

Chapter 4 – Healing Always Comes

Chapter 5 – Test of Faith

Chapter 6 – Renew Your Mind

Salvation Prayer

Dedication

This book is dedicated first and foremost to my parents who have since gone on to be with the Lord. Many mountains I had to climb without them, but because they taught me how to be an overcomer, pushing through obstacles and never quitting, I am able to say, "I made it".

I thank my siblings who have stood by me every step of every battle. A support system like no other.

Most of all I dedicate this book to my husband, Scott, and our four beautiful children, Noah, Emily, Olivia, and Jonah. Scott, you are the love of my life, my soulmate handpicked for me by God. You are my strength. Without your support and encouragement, I could not have done these last two battles.

Noah, Emily, Olivia, and Jonah I am so proud of your faith in God. Thank you all for being an extension of me and helping whenever I needed.

The faith my family has in God is amazing. To call upon His name and know He hears and answers prayer. Thank you for always praying and believing.

To God I give all the praise and glory forever and forever. My Healer, my Comforter, my Provider.

Cancer Has Nothing On Me

Chapter 1
In The Beginning

The Battle Begins

When you think of childhood memories, what are some of the things that come to mind? Your best friends, family time, your favorite pet? Slowly over the years those memories start to fade. You try hard to remember the small, intimate details; but along the way you lose them. Some memories make you smile; some make you sad. If only we could go back and relive just one of our best memories.

For me I have a memory that will be with me forever. The memory is as vivid today as when I lived it at 10 years old. Though I try hard to erase it from my mind, it is one that is etched so deep, I cannot. A scar that cannot be erased.

At the beginning of fifth grade, my family moved from Edgeworth to Sewickley, PA. There are just a few miles between the connecting towns, but for me that meant a new school district and new friends. I was a frightened little girl, but my worst fear was yet to come.

In April 1974 I had come home from school with a pain in my side. I told my mom, and like all moms she asked questions trying to figure out what I could have done. I was a very active child, a tomboy if you will. (My dad used to say he always thought he had three boys and one girl until I went to business school and started dressing like a girl.) My mom and I came to the conclusion I just hurt myself on the trampoline in gym class. I believed "our conclusion" and went to bed that night with no thought about it.

By morning, the pain was gone. As the weeks went on, I started losing weight and a lump formed on my stomach. I remember the day the pain came back. My brother and I were having a pillow fight and he hit me in the stomach. The pain came back with a vengeance that put me to my knees. If I laid, it hurt. If I sat, it hurt. If I breathed, it hurt. There seemed to be no relief. I had dropped weight to 54 pounds.

One day the pain was so intense that when my dad came home from work that night, my parents rushed me to the emergency room. After a few hours and a short visit with the ER doctor, we were sent home with a diagnosis of a pulled muscle. Within days the pain was gone. I was allowed back to gym class. I was back to being me.

By the end of the week, that horrific pain was back. I could not move from how bad it was. All I wanted to do was lay in bed. Again, my parents rushed me back to the ER. I remember my dad having to carry me to the car and into the ER because I could not walk. Again after a few hours and a second short visit by the same ER doctor, I was now diagnosed with having a bruised muscle. I was sent home with no relief.

As the pain grew worse and with no relief in sight, my mom made a doctor's appointment with our pediatrician. I was so afraid sitting in the doctors waiting room. I hung on to my mom's arm, hiding behind it. I didn't want to be there.

With an extensive exam, blood work and x-rays, I was quickly admitted to the hospital and scheduled for surgery. The hospital gown swallowed up my tiny body as I laid in the hospital bed that felt like a queen size bed to me. At 10 years old, I was confused, scared, and sad.

Staying Focused

What was this lump everyone was talking about? Why did I have to stay in the hospital? Why did I have to be alone? At 10 years old, it was a lot to take in for a little girl. I knew I wanted to be home with my family. I knew I wanted to be at school. I knew I wanted to be back home in my own bed. The one thing I did not know was the seriousness of what was going on. Fear had overtaken me. When my family left the hospital at night, I was alone and scared. How I cried for my parents and my life to be normal again.

After surgery, I remember waking up in the Intensive Care Unit, hooked to all the tubes, all the beeping machines and the little yellow duck on a shelf bobbing its head up and down. That little duck was my focus for the next week. It made me smile. If I could have just touched it, that would have made me happy. When nighttime came and the room was quiet, I focused on that little duck bobbing sitting on the shelf, out of my reach. The most important thing I remember of the ICU was my mom and dad right beside me, waiting for me to wake up. When I saw them, I knew I would be okay. During my stay in the hospital Intensive Care, God gave me a friend. Back in the 70's you didn't have your own room in the ICU. From what I can remember It was a big room separated by curtains. When the curtains were open, I talked with my new friend, Joe. Joe was an older man so gentle and kind. He was there because he was in a motorcycle accident and was having kidney problems. He and his wife became my comforters when my parents had to leave at night. He was my angel sent by God.

Diagnosed with a 10-pound tumor growing on my back, I had a long recovery ahead of me, but I knew, if I had my mom and dad, I would be okay and back to school before I knew it. Parents have a way of fixing things, and as a child, I thought they could fix this too.

Days turned into weeks which to me seemed like eternity. Finally, I was discharged from the hospital. All the nurses who had cared for me were there to say goodbye. One particular nurse became very special to me. Every day she would come in and see me. She had such a sweet spirit and was always smiling. Later I found out she was our neighbor. As a new friend, she always seemed to be watching out for me. Another angel God had placed in my life.

The doctor appointments that followed my surgery seemed never ending. The one I will forever remember is the last visit to Allegheny General Hospital. The Oncologist told my parents all the cancer had been removed. Not knowing if it was benign or malignant, they said no chemo was needed. After 54 days of missed school, I was released to return to a 10-year-olds life. I was thrilled!

Returning to school was not as easy as I thought. I met a friend when I transferred to the new school. When I was hospitalized, I thought she would forget about me; but she didn't. She became my best friend for the next six years. She was there for me as I was going through my ordeal. Along with her was a handful of other friends who would stop after school to visit with me while I was recovering. I was excited when I learned I could return to school and be with them.

The welcome back was wonderful. Everyone was so excited to have me back, but a few. I was new to all of them again. I let those few kids who were not excited to see me back make me feel like I was an outsider. One boy told me to go back where I came from because no one liked me. For years that one boy made me feel ugly and unwanted. I remember walking away from him and crying. I let him do that to me. That one negative statement stayed with me for years.

Praying Parents

As a mother of four healthy adults, I know the power of prayer. From the day we knew I was pregnant, and with each pregnancy after, I always prayed over our unborn children. Time and time again that has proven to be the only way our children survived the pregnancy. I had no idea that you could pray over an unborn child and have God protect it. I thought if I was protected, my child was protected.

From a lack of God's knowledge in protection, we lost our first child, Shannon. When we lost her, we were devastated. When we were told we would never have children and then Shannon was conceived, we knew it was a miracle. When we lost her, I did not understand; but if you will listen, God has a way to help you understand.

When we conceived Noah, our second pregnancy, we prayed protection for me and our unborn child. Every morning when I awoke and every night before I went to bed, I prayed over my Noah. This proved to be so vital as the pregnancy progressed and he was born 4 weeks early and not breathing. The reason I tell you all of this is to show the importance of praying for your children. I pray daily over my children to this day. The prayers of a mother are heard by God. God has answered those prayers in so many ways and in ways I do not even know.

It does not matter how you were raised. My mom was Orthodox and my dad Catholic. God hears your prayers when you cry out to him. During my cancer ordeal, God heard the prayers of my parents for protection and healing power. They cried out, and God heard and answered. Little did I know the impact their prayers and God's answer would have in my life. As a child, I trusted in my parents that they would take care of me and fix my broken little body. I knew the prayers of my parents were bombarding heaven, and God was not only hearing them, but meeting them where their faith was and answering those prayers.

Child-like Faith

It took me quite a long time to grasp the meaning of "child-like faith". One day during my quiet time with God, I picked up a book I was reading and came across this profound definition of child-like faith.

Child-like faith: A faith that does not doubt, question, or seek an explanation. It just believes. It is joyful. It goes boldly to the one you think can fix things. It is trusting and innocent.

This is the perfect description of me at 10 years old. I believed my parents could fix everything that went wrong or fix me when I was sick. They were my parents, and that is what parents do. They make everything right. At 10 years old, I needed my parents to fix me. I hung on so tight to my mom and dad, and they never let me go. As I hung on to them, they hung on to God.

Looking back now, I can see God answering their prayers to "fix me". To protect me. To heal me. It was a hope in the living God who can fix everything and anything that needs fixing.

Looking at my life now, I can see God answering my prayers and theirs asked in child-like faith.

Vivid Memory

Cancer? What was this cancer? Do other people get cancer? At such a young age, I had no idea the seriousness of what cancer was. To me this part of my life was over. I would never have to go through this again; or so I thought.

My memories of this trying experience are with me always because of the physical scar I wear. Cut open from one side of my belly to another, I always have the reminder of how God answered the cries of my parents to heal their daughter. Life's memories will slowly fade, but this one I cannot escape. God took a bad situation and turned it around for His glory and purpose. When bad things happen, God can use them to accomplish good (Romans 8:28 – And we know that all things work together for good to them that love God). Little did I know the true meaning of this.

Chapter 2
When God Meets You

Bad Thing Turned Good

Did you ever do something you know is bad or can hurt you but did it anyway? Of course you did! We all have. You think to yourself, "Oh, it will be alright. God will protect me." Can I tell you a tidbit of truth? If you step out from under God's umbrella of protection, He cannot protect you. It is just like if your parents tell you not to touch the hot stove and you do it anyway. They told you not to do it, but you wanted to. They tried to protect you but could not. You did it knowing there would be a consequence to pay, but at the same time thinking, "It will be ok. It won't hurt you".

God does not put anything bad on anyone ((Psalm 16:2 All good things come from God), but if you choose to do something you know is not right or going to hurt you, you are putting yourself in a dangerous situation. It's the thief that comes to kill, steal, and destroy (John 10:10), and he certainly was trying to steal my life.

At 25 years old, I took that step. For several years I stepped out from under God's umbrella, and it brought harm to me.

This step caused me great grief and is two-fold.

The first part of the two-fold was fear. Faith and fear cannot coexist. When I got into my teens, I had a secret fear that haunted me daily. I started smoking at 15 years old, and for years I had a fear of "what if". I had this fear that smoking would cause me cancer. I lived with the fear that I would have stomach cancer just like my dad. I lived that fear daily, but never heeded to the voice in me telling me to stop. I know today it was the voice of God trying to lead me back under His umbrella of protection. I ignored it. At the age of 25, the fear of cancer became a reality.

The second part of the two-fold was sickness. I was out from under God's protection for so long and living the devil's gift of fear, it manifested into stomach cancer. My fear became a reality. God did not put sickness on me. Had I listened to the Holy Spirit, had I not thought I was untouchable, I would have never set myself up to facing off with round two of cancer.

Receiving My Salvation

At 10 years old, I knew there was a God, but I knew nothing about this God. I thank my ex-mother-inlaw for her leading me to Christ. I wanted what she had. She loved Jesus and was not afraid to show it. She believed His Word, she worshiped freely with her amazing voice and shared salvation with whomever would listen.

At 18 I listened and was set free in a way I cannot even tell you. I accepted Jesus as my Lord and Savior. (Romans 10:9 If you declare with your mouth, "Jesus is Lord," and believe in your heart that God raised him from the dead, you will be saved.) From that point on, I wanted to know about my Jesus and His Word. That still small voice that spoke to my spirit long ago, I was starting to listen to. I started turning back to the safety of God's umbrella.

"Meet me, Lord"

"Meet me, Lord!" was my cry. When I passed blood one night In December 1987. I knew something was not right. That was my only indication of anything going on in my body . Once again, fear gripped my heart. I was trying to trust God, but I was losing the battle. Fear had a firm hold on me.

At 25, I was beyond the years of a pediatrician, but I called the doctor who discovered my first tumor, and he agreed to see me. Again, after an extensive exam, blood work and x-rays, I was told a tumor was consuming the bottom half of my stomach, engulfing four of the five layers of the stomach and two nodules were growing on my left lung.

This time I was alone. Sitting in the doctor's office listening to all he was saying was overwhelming. At one point I saw his lips moving but heard no sound. My head was spinning, my heart started racing and the fear slipped in so quickly I had hardly noticed. He gently hugged me as I sobbed on his shoulder. He told me, "We will get through this", and I believed him.

When I got home, I walked into the kitchen. My mom was standing at the kitchen sink, my dad sitting in his chair at the table and my sister and brother were in the dining room. I remember collapsing in one of the dining room chairs with my head in my hands crying uncontrollably. My brother walked over to me and just hugged me. I remember crying to him, "What am I going to do? Why?" I knew my siblings were in this with me and things were going to be okay. Once again fear had a grip on my mind and emotions.

Spiritually this time it was on me. I was at the age of accountability. I was an adult. What happened from here was on me. My mom and dad were there to cry with me and be there, but this time they could not fix me.

Over the next few weeks, I was referred to a surgeon. My mom was right there with me at the first appointment of many. Sitting in the waiting room I felt like that 10-year-old little girl again. I now understood cancer, and it scared me out of my mind. This time I could not hide behind my mom.

Meeting my surgeon for the first time I immediately felt at peace with him. He was such a kind and compassionate man. When he told me he had not stopped thinking of me for the last two weeks, I felt this was a man I wanted on my side. I became a name to him and not just a number. He was gentle with the whole cancer conversation reassuring me we would get through this. There were those words again.

The one question I asked him was, "Will I live long enough to see my kids?" He looked at me, smiled, and said, "Yes". For some reason, I felt a peace. I trusted his "Yes". Two weeks later I was scheduled for surgery.

The night before surgery, I laid in bed trying to find scriptures and hang on to a hope I knew nothing about. I remember praying to God to guide the hands of the doctors and nurses in the operating room. I remember begging Him to heal me; a healing that was already mine, but I did not know. When I cried out to God, "Meet me, Lord", He was faithful and met me where my faith was at. At 10 I had no faith. Now at 25 I had little faith, but my heart was not full of God's Word. I had to go with what I knew and that was God was a good God.

The surgeon's plan was to remove half of my stomach and the portion of my left lung with the nodules. As they were operating, a pathologist was running his tests. They had discovered there were cancer cells surrounding the stomach and opted for 80% of the stomach, finally taking 100% of the stomach "just to be safe". To open the chest and remove the portion of the lung would have been too much, so they left the lung and sewed me up. Filleted like a fish from breastbone to pelvic, I now had a vertical scar. Whenever I look at those scars, I see a sign of the cross reminding me God is always with me.

Knowing those nodules were still in me, drove me crazy. I later came to find out they had been calcified anywhere from 5 to 10 years. They were just sitting there. I had a doctor tell me that they have no clue why my body calcifies tumors; but it does. I know that only God can do something like that.

Waking up from surgery with all the tubes and beeping machines, I awoke to my mom, dad, sister, and brother there again by my side. My dad wiping away my tears as his own tears were streaming down his. Again, the prayers they bombarded heaven with were answered. To see them go through this again was painful for me. I felt I was the cause of their pain. When they cried, I cried. I did not cry for me this time. It was for them. My parents were the strongest people I will ever know. The next two weeks were hard weeks. This time the angel sent to me was my sister who never left my side.

She was there to cry with me, lift me up when I needed encouraged and fight the battle with me.

When I was transferred from ICU to a regular room, I shared that room with three different patients. The one woman I remember most was battling cancer herself. She was an older woman, and my heart went out to her. I tried everything I knew to witness to her. Telling her to trust God when I, myself, was trying to trust Him. My prayers went out for her. At night when the room was quiet and I could hear her faint breathing and her quiet groans of pain, I would pray for her asking God to please heal her. Eventually she was moved to a private room. As the days went by, I lost track of her, but my prayers for her remained.

The day after Christmas of 1987 I was discharged from the hospital and on my way back home. Hard days awaited me, but my cries to God were heard, and He was faithful. Just like how I hung on to my parents when I was 10, I now learned to hang on to God. I knew He would fix me. In John 10:10 He tells us that He came that we may have life and hive it abundantly. I was determined to have and abundantly, healthy life.

God created the human body with the ability to heal itself. And I was going to find out how.

I love to eat but eating became my biggest hurdle. With no stomach I could only eat a tablespoon of anything to begin with. Sometimes that would be too much, and I would get sick. It was a struggle to eat. It was a sow process, and even till this day meals are sometimes a challenge.

At 97 pounds, my agenda was to get back to normal and do the things I did before I got sick. As hard as it was on me sometimes, I pushed until I made it. I never gave up. Had I of given up I would have lost the battle. Cancer was not going to get the best of me, and it did not.

After surgery it was almost impossible to stand straight. I would stand against a wall with my arms stretched up over my head trying to stand as tall as I could. A physical challenge I eventually won. I fought so hard mentally, emotionally, and physically. Only God could have given me the strength I had to get through it.

At my next doctors visit, I was told the cancer was malignant and I would need chemo to try and shrink the nodules on my lung. Once again fear became my closest friend. I woke up in fear, lived the day in fear and went to bed with the same fearful, tormenting thoughts. I tried to hard to find the kind of faith that I knew I needed but fear always won.

The stomach cancer I was diagnosed with was so rare, the doctors could not find it in medical history. The morning I was scheduled to leave for Bethesda, Maryland for chemo treatments, the hospital called my Oncologist and said, "Do not send her. We do not know how to treat it." The doctors had discussed options over the phone on how to treat me. The method chosen was to admit me to the hospital, and chemo would run through my veins five days straight.

The morning I was hooked up to the chemo pump for my first round, I watched as the brownish medicine slowly started dripping into the long tube connected to the needle which now became one with me. Slowly, drip, drip, drip, pause. Again drip, drip, drip, pause. Finally, the chemo meds reached my hand and started flowing into my veins. I cried. I wanted to rip out the needle and run. Feeling like I was just issued a death sentence, all my mom could do for me was hug me and cry with me.

For the next week I was held captive to a drug which was worse than the cancer. I was so out of it from the drugs. I remember going into the hospital and coming back home. I have no memory of the five days in between.

Within two weeks of the first treatment, I lost my hair, eyebrows, and most of my lashes. I was devastated; but I was alive and getting through it. When I started losing my hair, it would come out in handfuls.
Oh, how I cried. As I look back now it was a vain thing. I thought my hair defined me. I remember the night I was with my sister in her room. I pulled my hair back and cut it all off. I felt like I lost me.

In the midst of all of this, I had started a new job. They had hired me the first week of December right before I got sick. I now had to explain to them I was diagnosed with stomach cancer. Surprisingly, they agreed to keep the position open for me, and when I was ready to come work for them, I could. So, I did. I lived with a bottle of Maalox in my desk drawer. Days were hard and long, but they worked with me even during the chemo. What a blessing that company was. This time it was a legion of angels given to me to help me get through the battle.

I started my first chemo treatment in January. A month later, I did my second treatment. The hair loss, the weight loss, the sickness; mentally it was just too much for me to handle another treatment. My emotions were all over the place. I would find myself crying for no reason other than I just didn't want to do it anymore. At the next visit with my Oncologist, I told him I was done. No more chemo. We argued over the whole decision, but he agreed to honor my wishes against his medical judgement. It was my choice.

For the next six years I saw my Oncologist every six months. Everything remained stable with no change. Six years turned into 20. I was cancer free. Any tumor in my body had calcified. I was home free or so I thought…again.

Chapter 3
Why Again?

Midlife Crisis

At midlife, what did you think, are thinking, or planning once you get there? A new car, a new job, a new home?

I was living the life! My kids were now 16, 14 and the twins 12. I was so enjoying my husband and kids. I loved my job. I loved my house. I was not having a midlife crisis. I had everything I wanted. I was doing everything I wanted to do. Life was so busy; I did not have time to stop and think half of the time.

I Never Asked, "Why Me?"

When the pains started in my gut, my first thought was, "I don't have time for this!". They would come and go lasting only for a short time. Then they started coming more frequently, staying just a little while longer each time. I started losing weight and feeling more tired. I wrote it all off to a busy life of working full-time, taking care of my house, and chasing four kids.

Every morning I would wake up there was no

pain. As the day progressed, I could feel the pain slowly coming on. As the day crept by, it got worse. Sometimes they were so crippling, I could not stand straight up. By the time I got home from work, the pain was unbearable. My family would scatter like mice when I walked into a room. No one wanted to be near me. There were nights I would go to bed at 7:00 p.m. with my bottle of Tylenol and heating pad praying for the pain to just leave.

In the midst of a full life, I was job searching. I felt stuck in a job that did not see my value. A job that I knew would always give me more work but never more pay. It was time to make a move, and I did. I found a job and was eager to start. When I started this new job, I wanted to learn and was willing to put my whole self into it; but there were some days I just could not concentrate. The pains were becoming more frequent and intense, staying a little longer each time.

I came home from work one night, and the pains were so bad. I sat on my bed rocking back and forth. There was no relief, no getting away from it. Somewhere around 10:00 p.m. I told my husband I could not take the pain anymore. I needed relief. He would not take no for an answer and off to the emergency room we went.

As with everything, when you take the step to see a doctor, the pain goes away. I wanted to go back home, but there was no going home that night. At around 1:00 a.m. I was admitted to the hospital scheduled for emergency surgery the next morning to remove the blockage in my intestine.

When things got bad, the first place I would run to was my mom. This time I couldn't. As I laid in the emergency room, she laid three floors up fighting her own health battle. My mom, my best friend, my support was losing her battle, and I couldn't even fix or help her. I felt my weakest in so many ways. The one thing I could do was pray for her. I knew God had her, and that gave me the inner strength to fight the battle I was facing.

This time I was standing as me; the woman she had birthed, raised, and instilled values in. The strength she showed in life taught me more than she could have ever imagined. Watching her push through whatever life handed her helped and continues to help me get through what I face. She will always be my hero.

When I awoke from the surgery and was coherent enough to understand, I was told I had stage 4 colon cancer which had metastasized. I was also told a foot of my colon was removed, but they did get all the cancer. Because the intestines were so inflamed, they had no choice but to give me a temporary colostomy. Working in DME I knew what people with a colostomy dealt with, and I never wanted to be one of them. Yet here I was. I name the colostomy "Tomas" (stoma). I refused to say, 'my colostomy or stoma". It was only temporary, and as soon as I got my second clear scan, Tomas was gone!

What a whirlwind of emotions. The one questions I never asked God was, "Why me?" I did ask, "Why again?"

Three Strikes And Still Standing

The first thoughts that bombarded my mind were not good. Thoughts of death haunted me day and night. What was my husband going to do? How were my kids going to grow up without their mom? I fought hard to erase those thoughts from my mind. I hardly waited to get home from the hospital to be with my family. These days hospitals kick you out right away. I wasn't going to argue. I wanted to be home.

Once home, I did fine during the day. Scott would leave for work, and I would drop the kids off to school. I did what I needed to do for my family. At night was the hardest. As soon as my door was shut, the tears would start. I would drop to my knees and beg God for things I do not even remember. I just wanted to live.

One night I was going up to bed, and I was halfway up the steps when Scott said to me, "The Lord assured me you would not die, but live and declare His works." I knew this was a promise of God found in Psalm 118:17. I knew if God spoke this to Scott, this was something He wanted me to know. My mind was racing so fast, I could not hear God. I believed God spoke this to Scott not just for him but for me. I received this scripture as my own.

    That night when I got in bed, the racing in my mind had slowed down. I now took that one scripture and started confessing it. As I started searching God's Word for promises on healing, the next profound scripture was, "With long life will I satisfy you and show you my salvation" Psalm 91:16. I was now double fisted with scripture. I took hold of those scriptures and confessed them until I think God got tired of hearing me. (Just to let you know, God never gets tired of hearing you.) He started opening my eyes to see the promises of healing. Healing was already mine. I had to receive it now.

    The mind is constantly going. It's always thinking of something whether it be positive or negative. To stop the negative thoughts, I would start confessing God's Word out loud so that I not only heard it, but the enemy heard it too. He whispers, but God speaks.

    With the cancer having metastasized, my Oncologist wanted to do chemo treatments to try and shrink the tumor in my chest. I now weighed in at 89 pounds. I agreed, and for the next six weeks chemo treatments were every other week. I would go in the office to receive an eight-hour treatment. Then they would hook me up to go home on a machine that would pump chemo for another 24 hours. I would go home and forget I was hooked to this machine so it ended up hitting the floor more times that I could count. At night I heard that constant breathing of the machine that reminded me it was with me. Hours seemed like days to me. When I was alone is when the negative thoughts would speak the loudest.

  Then started the neuropathy. It started out slow. I would have tingling in my hands, sensitivity to hot and hold and loss of feeling. When the feeling did not come back to my hands, the chemo medication was changed. At this point, the neuropathy was in my hands, feet and stopped at my knees. I was told the feeling would come back. As of today, eight years later, the neuropathy is still there. I can sympathize now with the people who have lived with this for years. It is not fun. I may not be able to feel things with my hands, but my hands still function, and my legs still walk me places. I can stand and declare the works of Jesus.

  As I sat there through every treatment, I would hear the people around me talking about their illness. Whose was worse? Who hurt more? Who could complain the most? I started losing my compassion for people. I would leave the office and just cry, "Lord, please! I cannot do this anymore."

Negativity breeds negativity. As I went through each treatment, God started showing me that these people are hurting just like me. They are looking for someone to listen to them, to sympathize with them. Then He started leading me to pray for them. My whole perspective of the chemo room started to change, and I found myself started feeling compassion for them. I would sit in the chair during treatment and look for people to pray for. People to just listen to. I was mentally exhausted when I left the chemo chair just listening to all the talk of sickness. I was doing what God wanted me to do so I knew he would give me the strength to get through it.

Leaving It At God's Feet

At the end of the six months of treatment, a scan showed the tumor was not shrinking. I was sent to a liver specialist who said that the type of cancer I had usually gives the patient up to 18 months from diagnosis. I still refused to accept the report of what the doctors were saying. I knew they couldn't do anything else for me; but God could. We thanked him for his time and left.

Going back to my oncologist with this information did not put a fear in me. I knew what God had spoken was my future. I would live a long life. I was not giving in to what the doctors were telling me. I chose to believe God's report over theirs. When it comes to fighting for your life, it does not matter what others think. They were not my problem.

My oncologist suggested "maintenance" chemo. It would hold the cancer at bay for a while, but there was no guarantee for how long. He did not want to open me back up to reverse the colostomy. Well, that was an argument waiting to happen. He made a promise I wasn't going to let me out of. I did the chemo and the scans. I was cashing in on that promise. According to God's Word, I was healed. I no longer need Tomas. It was time for him to leave.

At this point, only Scott and our four children knew what was going on. People outside of our circle knew I had cancer and knew I was taking treatments. No one ever knew how serious it was. As a family, we agreed we would not discuss it outside of our family, and we all prayed in one accord the promises of God. I told Scott I had enough and was not going to do the 'maintenance' chemo. He supported my decision.

As a family, we lifted it up to God and left it at His feet. Our trust was in Him. We prayed and then never spoke of chemo, cancer, or anything remotely close after that. I told my family no one is to treat me as if I am sick. I will continue to be mom and wife just like before. I wanted no special treatment, and believe me, I did not get it.

It is never too early to teach your kids God's Word. They knew at 16, 14 and 12 God could and would heal their mom. I promised them I was not going anywhere. They believed me, but most importantly, they believed God.

Chapter 4
The Answer Always Comes

I Never Travel Alone

There were days my body was so tired, so zapped of energy. I would see Scott off to work, drive the kids to school, then come home and collapsed. All my crying was done behind doors, alone with God. He had promised me in His Word that He would never leave me or abandon me. Every tear I cried, He cried with me. When I could not lift myself up, He carried me. I knew I was never alone.

As an adult I learned over the years to go to God with child-like faith. He is our Father, and we are his children. I have learned to pray the Word and not beg for it, to pray in faith and not fear and to pray the answer and not the problem.

God Knows Our Needs

God knows our needs before we even have the need, but how He responds is by faith, our faith.

Early on in my journey I had hope that God would move for me. I was always hoping for healing, hoping cancer would just go away, hoping cancer would never come back. It was not until I got a revelation on faith that I knew my hopes would be answered.

As I studied God's Word on faith, I learned an unshakeable confidence that commands and speaks with a boldness that cannot be denied. I have learned to speak over situations that have no choice but to change. Some things take longer than others, but if I stand my ground and never speak against my need, it has no choice but to manifest. Healing always comes. You must know the moment you are prayed for you are healed. Then you must be willing to stand until you see the manifestation. You must hold on like a dog on a bone. Never giving into feelings or what you see. Praising God for the answer before you see it.

You cannot rehydrate from an empty well. If there is nothing left in the well, where do you pull water from? It is the same with your spirit. If you find yourself in a situation you cannot get yourself out of, what do you do? That is when the fear sets in. The complaining starts. You start dropping faith hints to people hoping they catch what you are dropping, and they will help you. That is not faith. Faith is walking through the test with a smile on your face knowing God has your answer, and the answer will not be late.

On the other hand, if you fill your spirit up on God's promises before any situation arises, as soon as a sickness tries to come upon you, you can stop it in Jesus' name. You can speak the Word of God regarding your situation whether it be a financial need, healing, forgiveness of sin, joy, peace, and the list goes on. You can take your rightful place as a child of God and speak with a faith that commands with boldness and confidence knowing what He has spoken will come to pass.

It's Always Something

Early on in my Christian walk I always thought, "I'm a Christian! I'll never have to face any problems because I am God's." How wrong I was. God never said we would not have tests or trials, but He did tell us how to handle them. James 1:2-4 tells us to count it all joy when we are met with trials… the testing of our faith produces steadfastness. 1Peter 4 tells us not to be surprised at the fiery trials "when" they come. 1Cor 10:13 says that with the temptation he will also provide the way of escape.

There are many more scriptures regarding tests and trials, but the end is always the same, God has the way out. When a test or trial comes, and they will, do not complain, do not blame God. Stretch your faith and let God provide the way of escape.

Whose Report Will You Believe?

I can see over the years how my believing has progressed from doubt to belief, hope to faith. When I had my first cancer battle, the only report I was concerned about was a report I was doing on Kentucky in school. (The simple things you remember surrounding a traumatic event.)

When faced with my second cancer battle, I knew more of God's Word. I started believing God would meet me at my faith. When I heard the report of the doctors, fear gripped me hard; but I knew God would meet me where my faith was. I prayed He would guide the hands of the doctor who gave me the report I would live to see my kids and was declared cancer free. He met me at what I could believe for.

The report given me by doctors during my third cancer battle was not good. I had a decision to make. Either I was going to believe what the doctors were saying and give up on life or I was going to believe the report of God who said, "By my stripes you were healed." I had a choice to make. This time there was no question on whose report would I believe. I knew what God had promised, and I knew the promise was mine. Was it an easy battle? Not always. But I renewed my mind with the Word of God daily. I fed on His Word until the doubt and fear left. My mind was so convinced that I was healed, sometimes I forgot I was battling. Not only did I have to fight against doubt and fear but also against the conversations with friends who looked at me like I was deathly ill (at times I was), people talking about you when you were in a room, and people feeling sorry for me. I knew if I gave in to the sympathy I would have stayed there. Sometimes it was hard to push through when I wanted to give up.

I told God I did not want to die yet. I wanted to raise my kids and hold my grandbabies. I wanted to travel with my husband and share the gospel with anyone who would listen. I needed Him, and I knew He would not fail me.

So, when you feel your weakest and sickest, do not give up. Choose whose report you will believe and stay with that report. Do not waiver. God is not holding anything back from you. His will for healing is in His Word.

Having Done All To Stand…Stand!

Stand firm! Hold your ground! Speak the Word! There will be times when you feel you are losing the battle. If you are standing on the Word of God for healing, those feelings of losing are just that, feelings. When you think you just cannot go on and God will not help you, you can, and He will.

When you say, "I've tried all those scriptures, and they aren't working." One thing I can tell you is you do not "try" God's Word. You either believe it or not. You cannot try it.

When you catch yourself speaking contrary to what you are believing, you can go to God and ask Him to forgive you for doubting. Just get back in the Word and press on. Faith is of the heart not the head. What you speak about your situation is what you have filled your heart with. (Matt 12:34 Out of the abundance of the heart the mouth speaks.)

The Answer Always Comes

Ironically, 47 years after I began my journey, I just came to find out the name of the cancer I had was "Carney Triad". Coincidence? Maybe. I know that I know, no matter the name medical science calls it, God calls it cursed, dissolved, rebuked. So, what is my heart full of? My heart and head are convinced, because of God and His wonderful promises of healing, cancer has nothing on me.

Chapter 5
Test Of Faith

The Thorn In My Side

Cancer is the thorn in my side. I believe in my spirit this is its last attempt to put me under. After eight years of cancer lying dormant, it has once again reared its ugly head. At my yearly scan in November 2020, the one growth my Oncologist has been watching, grew one centimeter. When I got the call from him, I was not concerned. Then I got the devastating news; he is retiring. My heart sunk!

Since 1987 he has been the one doctor who has always had my back. He has seen me at my best, and he has seen me at my worst. He was always willing to hear my side of things and always ready for my debates.

When he told me in 2014 chemo was not helping and I called it quits, he stood by my decision: not once, but twice. When I heard he was retiring, I gave in this time. I agreed to do things his way. What a blessing that decision turned out to be.

For a quick recap, I had cancer at ages 10, 25 and 49 and now at 57. Since my doctor is retiring, I agreed to all the tests he wanted to do. The endless bloodwork, CT scans, colonoscopy, mammogram, and biopsy of the tumor.

Through Thanksgiving, Christmas, New Years and Serbian Christmas, Scott and I managed to keep it all hush-hush. As my Oncologist spoke with the pathologist and radiologist, he was getting closer to diagnosing this type of tumor. He worked endlessly for me, finally finding a doctor at the Hillman Cancer Center who specializes in what they thought this tumor was. With more blood work and a dotatate scan, it was confirmed. The type of cancer that has invaded my body all these years is Paraganglioma. With a two in one million chance of getting this, I drew one of the two chances.

I told my doctors the two things I did not want was surgery, (11 surgeries were enough) and chemo. Before the dotatate scan there was a chance of a treatment that was not a chemo. Unfortunately, that hope was short lived. Insurance denied my one chance of no chemo. Here I was again faced with chemo.

Treatments started and were to be every three weeks for four treatments. They were a two-day treatment leaving me drained of energy and sick to my stomach. After three weeks I was at the point where I could not do it anymore. My doctor agreed to a CT scan which showed chemo wasn't doing anything. Chemo, once again, was stopped.

What is next? I'm not sure yet. Leading up to the last treatment, I felt a whole lot of "I'm not sure what". I never got angry, fearful, or anxious. I have a peace that only comes from God. He will direct my path and will tell me what I need to do next.

The Testing of Your Faith

I know this is another test of my faith. Trials come, but I know, so does God. He even tells us in His word how to overcome them.

1Peter 1:7 tells me These trials are only to test your faith, to whether or not it is strong and pure. My faith is certainly being tested. Through the years I have filled my heart up with only God's promises. So, yes, my faith is being tested but it is now strong enough to walk through the battle untouched.

Deuteronomy 8:2 And you shall remember that the Lord your God led you all the way these 40 years in the wilderness, to humble you and test you, to know what is in your heart, whether you would keep His commandments. I have certainly been humbled in so many different ways. By the words I speak in or out of a test, you can tell what is in my heart. You yourself can tell what is in your own heart. Listen to the words you speak.

James 1:3 count it all joy when you fall into various trials…. the testing of your faith.

Chapter 6
Renew Your Mind

Renew Your Mind

Romans 12:2 And be not conformed to this world; but be ye transformed by the renewing of your mind, that you may prove what is that good, and acceptable, and perfect, will of God.

Faith takes work. You cannot believe in something you do not know. When you are under attack of any kind, the mind will gravitate toward the negative. To build your faith, you must daily renew your mind with the Word of God. It will not happen overnight, but with constantly renewing your mind you will get it in your heart, and when an attack of the enemy comes, you will be able to reach down and grab God's Word that has been planted. You will be able to speak to the mountain and watch as God removes it.

You can have great faith, little faith, or no faith. What you put into it is what you get out. Heb 11:6 says, "But without faith it is impossible to please him; for he that comes to God must believe that He is, and that He is a rewarder of those who diligently seek Him". I wanted the kind of faith that pleased God. So, the more I spoke the Word of God the more I was hearing, hearing,

hearing. Are you hearing me? You must keep the Word in front of and in you.

Daily I would confess: The Spirit of God is upon me. The healing power of God is within me working in my body to perfect a healing and a cure. No tumor can successfully grow in my body. They are dissolved in my body, and I am whole and healthy.

No matter how I felt, my words never changed. I rebuked sickness and disease. I spoke to aches and pains commanding them to leave my body in Jesus' name. I only spoke life. Once I knew in my heart God would heal me, healing is all I spoke. It did not matter how I felt inside. It did not matter what I looked like outside. I just knew if God said I was healed then I was healed.

God's Word says in Proverbs 29:18 Where there is no vision, the people perish. In Habakkuk 2:2 it says, "Write the vision and make it plain on tablet, that he may run who hears it". I did not want to die. I wanted to be whole and healthy, so I wrote down in my journal how I wanted to feel, how I wanted to look and all that I wanted to accomplish. Daily I would thank God for the answer to that vision. I never said I was sick, only healthy and strong. I would never say I can't. I did everything I set my mind to. I told myself I can, I will and I am. One other favorite scripture of mine was and still is, "I can do all things through Christ who strengthens me" Philippians 4:13. Quitting was not an option.

I never confessed God's Word to one person and to the next, complain. You might as well spit in the wind because everything you confess is nullified when you speak contrary to what you are believing for. You cannot ride the fence and expect to see results.

If you read through the Gospels (Matthew, Mark, Luke, and John) you will never find a situation that Jesus was not willing to heal someone. He healed all. Some immediately, some the selfsame hour, some from that hour. He healed them all, limbs were restored, as many as were touched were made whole (Matthew 14:36)! What are you in need of today? God will do the same for you!

Praying and Praising

The two P's that work hand-in-hand are pray and praise. I said earlier I was starting to lose the compassion for people every time I sat in the chemo chair. All they wanted was to complain and compare. In subsequent chemo treatments during my last battle, God showed me people are not looking to complain or compare (though there are those who look to do just that), they are looking for someone to listen. I told the Holy Spirit, "Use me".

I will listen, but I will not participate in the complaining or comparing.

As I listened to the stories my heart started to hurt for these people. If only they knew about my God. The Holy Spirit told me one day to start sharing what I knew. How I got healed. How I got through the pain and sickness. How I found joy. Little by little I did just that. I started praying for those people. I did not know their names, but God did. He knew what they needed. I was just a vessel He could use. If you have nothing to say, pray. Prayers will move mountains.

As time went on and the people were getting their chance to ring the last chemo treatment bell, I found myself now praising God for answers to prayers I had prayed. Through sources I learned some of those people won their battle. Some sadly did not. For that short period of time, I got to spend with them, some of the complaining had stopped, and I could see a ray of hope.

When you pray according to the Word of God, there is nothing left to do but praise your way until you see your manifestation. God is not a liar. What He has promised will come to pass. Just have faith and never quit. When you can praise God in the midst of a trail is when you know you truly believe your answer is coming.

Scriptures That Helped Me Win The Battle

Psalm 91:14-16 Because he hath set his love upon me, therefore will I deliver him: I will set him on high, because he hath known my name. 15He shall call upon me, and I will answer him: I will be with him in trouble, I will deliver him, and honor him. 16With long life will I satisfy him and shew him my salvation.

Sometimes you can be so confused and scared you just cannot hear God if He were standing in front of you. That is when God will use someone else to get the message to you. When God spoke this to Scott, that is the night my healing took place. I needed a wakeup call, and God gave it. I am so thankful Scott is sensitive to the Holy Spirit.

Psalm 118:17 I shall (will) not die, but live, and declare the works of the Lord.

When the Holy Spirit spoke this to me, I received it. The Bible never tells us we will be test free. We are told in James 1:12 Blessed is the man who perseveres under trial, 1Peter 4:12 Do not be surprised at the painful trial you are suffering. The Bible does tell us tests and trials are coming. It also tells us how to handle them. God has given you the answer to every problem you will ever face. Read your Bible.

Jeremiah 30:17 For I will restore health unto thee, and I will heal thee of thy wounds.

God told me He will restore health to me and heal me of my wounds. He said it, I believe it.

Isaiah 53:5 But he was wounded for our transgressions, he was bruised for our iniquities: the chastisement of our peace was upon him; and with his stripes we ARE healed.

1Peter 2:24 Who his own self bore our sins in his own body on the tree, that we, being dead to sin, should live unto righteousness: by whose stripes you WERE healed.

I was healed, I am healed. What more do I need? Isaiah 53:5 and 1Peter 2:24 are also two of my favorite scriptures. I am covered in both the Old Testament with ARE and in the New Testament with WERE. In plain words… I was, I am, I will be!

Isaiah 54:17 No weapon formed against me shall (will) prosper.

There might be a weapon formed against me, but it will not prosper. Do not give it a chance. God said the weapon (of sickness, disease, depression, lack, whatever the weapon is) will NOT prosper.

1John 4:4 Ye are of God, little children, and have overcome them: because greater is he that is in you, than he that is in the world.

As a born-again believer, the Holy Spirit lives inside me. He is my strength when I need it. He is my peace, my joy, my hope. In Him I rest and know that the Spirit of God is upon me and the Holy Spirit lives in me. I am covered both in and out.

Mark 5:34 And he said unto her, Daughter, thy faith hath made thee whole, go in peace, and be whole of thy plague.

What is your faith speaking? Do you believe when you reach out and ask God for help that He will help? Are you asking in hope or faith? Faith in our living God gets answers.

Mark 5:36 Be not afraid, only believe.

Matthew 9:22 thy faith has made thee whole.

Matthew 9:29 According to your faith be it unto you.

What are you believing? Are you believing what the symptoms and your surroundings are saying or are you renewing your mind daily with the promises of God and believing what His Words says despite what you are dealing with?

Mark 11:23-24 For verily I say unto you, that whosoever shall say unto this mountain, Be thou removed and be thou cast into the sea; and shall not doubt in his heart but shall believe that those things which he saith shall come to pass; he shall have whatsoever he saith. 24Therefore I say unto you, what things soever ye desire, when ye pray, believe that you shall (will) have them.

What are you saying to your mountain? Are you giving it room to grow? Are you feeding it? Or are you removing the mountain?

Matthew 19:26 But Jesus beheld them, and said unto them, With men this is impossible, but with God all things are possible.

Healing always comes. The moment you are prayed for your healing is. Do not look at the circumstances. Stand Firm. The violent will take it by force. It is a spiritual battle, and believe me, the devil is real. He is trying his hardest to remove you from this world. There is no disease or sickness too big for our God. How bad do you want healed? Are you willing to fight the good fight?

Cancer is not a death sentence.

Salvation Prayer

Have you accepted Jesus as Lord and Savior of your life? If you die tomorrow, do you know where you will spend eternity. If not, pray this simple prayer and start a new life in Christ.

Father, I come to You in the Name of Jesus. I admit that I am not right with You, and I want to be right with You. I ask You to forgive me of all my sins. The Bible says if I confess with my mouth that "Jesus is Lord" and believe in my heart that God raised Him from the dead, I will be saved (Romans 10:9). I believe with my heart, and I confess with my mouth that Jesus is the Lord and Savior of my life. I invite you into my heart. Thank you for saving me. In Jesus' Name I pray. Amen

www.ingramcontent.com/pod-product-compliance
Lightning Source LLC
Chambersburg PA
CBHW051204170526
45158CB00005B/1810